Faten LIMAIEM

Practical Guide to Urological Pathology

Faten LIMAIEM

Practical Guide to Urological Pathology

Essential protocols

ScienciaScripts

Cover image: www.ingimage.com

This book is a translation from the original published under ISBN 978-620-6-69561-5.

Publisher:
Sciencia Scripts
is a trademark of
Dodo Books Indian Ocean Ltd. and OmniScriptum S.R.L publishing group

120 High Road, East Finchley, London, N2 9ED, United Kingdom
Str. Armeneasca 28/1, office 1, Chisinau MD-2012, Republic of Moldova, Europe
Managing Directors: Ieva Konstantinova, Victoria Ursu
info@omniscriptum.com

Printed at: see last page
ISBN: 978-620-8-63501-5

Practical Guide to Urological Pathology

Essential protocols

TABLE OF CONTENTS

FOREWORD

The macroscopic examination of urological surgical specimens is an essential step in the diagnostic and therapeutic process. This guide has been developed specifically for specialists in pathological anatomy, to assist them in the analysis of various surgical specimens, including pediatric nephrectomy, partial and total nephrectomy, excretory tract tumor surgery, as well as testicular specimens, radical prostatectomy and cystoprostatectomy.

Urological pathologies, particularly malignant ones, have distinctive morphological features that require special attention. The aim of this guide is to provide a clear methodology, with appropriate protocols, for the careful examination of these specimens. Each chapter is designed to facilitate tumor identification, precise description and evaluation of prognostic factors essential to patient management.

We hope that this tool will be a valuable ally in your training, helping you to develop the skills you need to excel in urological pathological anatomy. Wishing you every success in your studies and practice, we encourage you to approach each surgical specimen with rigor, curiosity and a spirit of critical analysis.

NEPHRECTOMY IN CHILDREN

NEPHRECTOMY IN CHILDREN

A- Anatomy - Orientation :

1. External view :

The kidney is bean-shaped, with two faces, anterior and posterior, medial and lateral, and upper and lower poles.

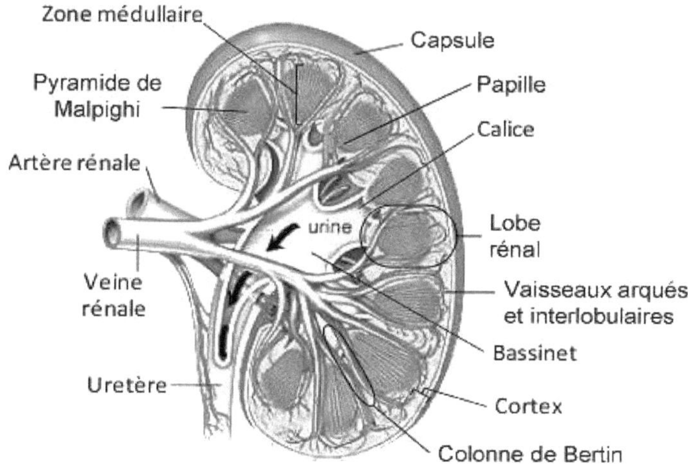

Figure 1: Schematic of a longitudinal kidney section (modified from M. Keck, 2012).

2. Longitudinal section :

Retroperitoneally located paired organ surrounded by a fibrous capsule, then by abundant adipose tissue bounded by Gerota's fascia (visible in surgery or radiology), penetrated by renal arteries and veins in the hilum at the medial edge.

- The renal parenchyma includes

  - **Peripheral cortex** with glomeruli and proximal and distal convoluted tubules

  - A **central medullary** with the coves of Henlé and collecting tubes. The collecting tubes terminate at the papilla in a minor calyx.

3. Urinary tract

Blood is filtered by the **glomeruli.** The glomerular ultrafiltrate (or primary urine) is modified as it passes through successive segments of the **nephrons**:

- proximal contour tubes of the cortex

- the Henle's loops of the medulla

- distal convoluted tubes of the cortex

- then into the medullary collecting tubes

The final urine then flows into the minor calyces.

The minor calyces form the beginning of the urinary tract. Urine collects in the **major calyces**, then in the **pyelon** (formerly the renal pelvis), which flows into **the ureter** at the lower end of the hilum. The ureter continues the extra-renal transport of urine into the **bladder** and **urethra**.

4- His reports :

- **Right kidney:**

- posterior side: diaphragm above, psoas, quadratus lumborum and transverse abdominis below.

- the visceral surface of the right lobe of the liver and duodenum on the upper anterior surface, and the right colonic angle on the lower surface.

- The liver runs along the lateral edge.

- medial edge, the right adrenal gland above, the renal hilum in the middle and the ureter below.

- **Left kidney:**

- posterior side: diaphragm above, psoas, quadratus lumborum and transverse abdominis below.

- anterior face above the spleen and tail of the pancreas, and in its middle and lower parts the jejunal ansae and left colonic angle.

- lateral edge of the left colonic angle.

- The left adrenal gland is on the medial edge, the renal hilum on the middle edge and the ureter on the lower edge.

5- Orientation criteria :

- **Adrenal**

Orange-yellow, at the upper pole of the kidney, extending over the upper part of the medial border.

- **In case of tumor:** (here upper pole) check if tumor location corresponds to clinical information

Renal hilum: medial

Ureter: Path from pyelon to lower pole

runs along the medial edge of the kidney to its lower pole.

Easily found before opening, its end corresponding to the lower-medial part of the kidney.

B- Measure, weigh and photograph the intact surgical specimen:

- Measuring

I__I__I__Ix I__I__I__Ix I__I__I__Imm

- Weighing

I__I__I__I__Igrams

- Take photographs, pinpointing areas of suspected breakage.

C- Encircling the surgical part :

- **Sponging** the surgical specimen

- **Encircling** the workpiece

- **Allow to** air **dry** for a few minutes, then **immerse the** workpiece in acetic formalin (rather than Bouin's liquid).

D- Open the operating room and photograph :

- **Sponging** the surgical specimen

- **Open the kidney** at its outer edge, trying to position yourself in the plane of the renal hilum.

E- Describe the lesion :

Number:I__I__I

- Size: I__I__I__Ix I__I__I__Ix I__I__Imm

- Location:

□ Upper fleece□ Medio-renal□ Hilaire□ Lower fleece□ Massive

- Assess the percentage of necrosis: I__I__I %.

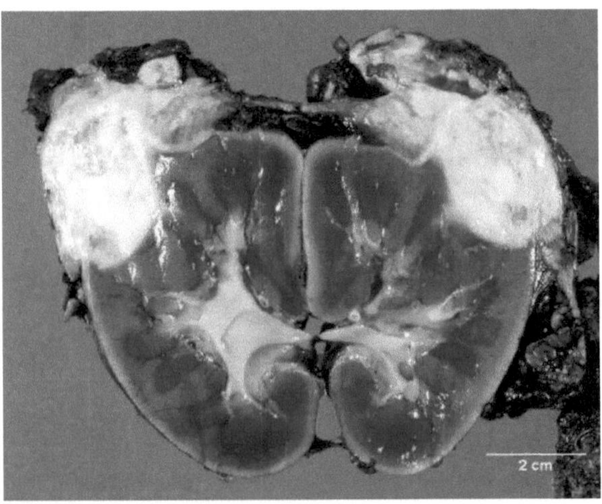

Figure 2: Soft, yellow-brown, lobulated tumour near the upper pole of the kidney. The tumour extends beyond the kidney and appears to be present on the inked surgical margin.

https://www.webpathology.com/images/genitourinary/kidney/pediatric-renal-tumors-i---nephroblastoma/36019

F- Securing the surgical part :

- **Formaldehyde** or acetic formaldehyde

The part can be placed at 4°C for better fixation

- Duration 24 to 48 hours

Fixation can be further accelerated by performing a slice parallel to the first one a few hours after surgery (the renal capsule no longer retracts as it did when the operating room was opened).

G- Sampling :

- **One or two complete slices of the tumor** passing through the hilum and, if possible, the longest axis of the tumor are included in their entirety and marked out, involving both the normal kidney and the tumor.

- The location of each sample must be indicated on the photograph (block numbering).

- **Additional sampling**

If necessary, on other suspicious areas, at the periphery of the tumour, at the level of the renal hilum, on normal kidney if this is absent from complete slices (take two blocks of normal kidney).

H- Look for sinus adenopathy:

- On palpation

- Include all lymph nodes found

I - Equipment

- Fixing agent: The usual fixing agent is 10% buffered formalin.
- blade
- Knife
- India ink
- Flat ruler
- Tapes
- Camera

J. Conditions and rules of good practice

- Parts are fixed in 10% buffered formalin.
- Delayed or poor fixation can alter the morphological quality of histological sections. It is important to respect the ratio of tissue volume to fixative volume (1/10).

- All specimens must be sent to the pathology laboratory together with a **clinical information sheet**. This sheet should include the history of the disease, the patient's background, the results of any paraclinical examinations carried out, and endoscopic data.

K. Conclusion

In conclusion, a methodical and accurate approach to the macroscopic examination of nephrectomy specimens is imperative to characterize tumor lesions, assess resection margins and provide crucial information for patient prognosis and management. By following the guidelines presented in this guide, pathology professionals will be able to perfect their ability to accurately interpret the macroscopic characteristics of tumors, thus contributing to more effective, individualized patient management.

What to sample

■ **2 macroscopic slices**

The blocks are marked on a photograph of the two macroscopic slices. At least 1 macroscopic slice.

■ **Normal kidney** (2 blocks) (if absent from both slices)

■ **Any other** suspicious **lesion(s)**

■ Any **lymph nodes** in the renal hilum

SIOP classification (International Society of Pediatric Oncology)

SIOP stages (pre-nephrectomy chemotherapy)

☐ No TNM classification for renal tumours in children but SIOP classification

☐ SIOP classification varies according to whether or not preoperative treatment has been performed.

☐ In France, children's kidney tumors are removed after chemotherapy

Stage 1

T must be completely resected (negative margins

a) Tumor limited to the kidney or surrounded by a fibrous pseudo-capsule that may be infiltrated by the tumor

b) Tumour protruding into the excretory tract or ureter, but must not infiltrate its wall

c) Necrotic tumor tissue, or post-chemotherapy remodeling in the sinus, but sinus vessels must be free of tumor and necrosis.

d) Tumor invading intra-renal vessels

Note: a transcutaneous fine-needle biopsy or aspiration does not change the stage (the needle size (Gauje) must be mentioned to the Pathologist).

Stage 2

a) Tumour extends into perirenal fat, but resection is complete (margins -)

b) Tumor infiltrates sinus or extra-renal vessels, but complete resection

c) Tumor infiltrates adjacent organs or vena cava, but complete resection

d) Surgical biopsy prior to surgery or chemotherapy

Stage 3

a) Incomplete tumour excision extending to the resection margins

b) Invasion of one or more abdominal lymph nodes

c) Pre- or intraoperative tumor rupture

d) Tumor penetrates the peritoneal surface

e) Tumor implants on the peritoneal surface

f) Tumor thrombi present in the vessel or ureter resection margins or sent fractionated by the surgeon

Note: the presence of tumour necrosis or chemotherapy-induced changes (foamy histiocytes) in a lymph node or resection margin is considered evidence of tumour.

Stage 4

Hematogenous metastasis (lung, liver, bone, brain, etc.) or lymph node metastasis outside the abdominal-pelvic region

Stage 5

Bilateral tumor at diagnosis

If in doubt about tumor stage, refer urgently to referral pathologist.

PARTIAL NEPHRECTOMY

PARTIAL NEPHRECTOMY

A- Orienting the part :

- Locate the outer surface of the kidney (smooth lining (capsule) or adipose tissue)
- Any other marking (top/bottom...) is usually impossible in the absence of a surgical marker.

B- Measuring, weighing and inking :

- **Measuring** the surgical excision fragment

I__I__I__Ix I__I__I x I__I__I mm

- **Weigh** the communicated fragment

I__I__I__Igrams

Only if the part arrives intact (unopened by the surgeon)

- The parenchymal surgical resection zone

- The external surface of the tumor if there is no fat.

C- Opening the room :

In its longest axis from its outer edge, perpendicular to the inked surgical section

D- Describe the tumor :

- **Measuring** the tumor ↔

I__I__I__Ix I__I__I x I__I__I mm

- **Contours**

□ well limited□ poorly limited

□ encapsulated□ non-encapsulated

- Consistency

□ farm□ molle

□ buff yellow□ light beige

□ mahogany brown□ polychrome other

- Reshuffles

□ necrotic: |__|__| %.

□ bleeding□ scarring

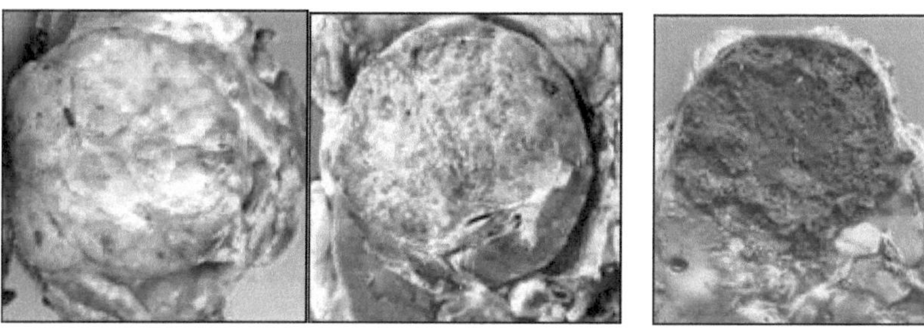

Chamois yellow Light beige Mahogany brown

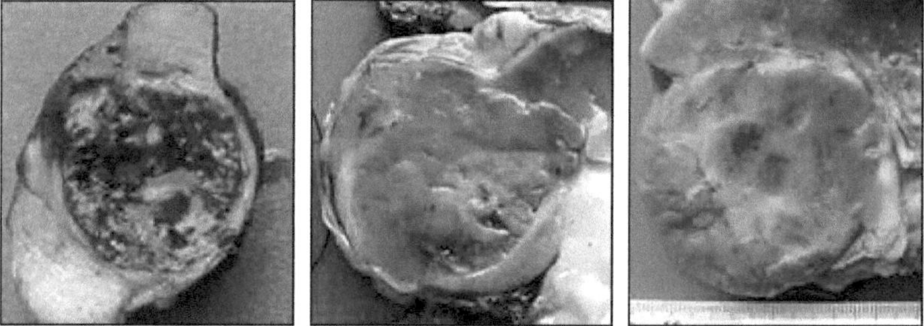

Polychrome Dark beige Orange yellow

E- Specify ratios, measure them

- Infiltration of the renal capsule

□ yes

□ no (margin : I__I__I mm) (1 block)

□ absent (no renal capsule)

- Infiltration of fat

□ yes (depth I__I__I mm)

□ no (margin : I__I__I mm) (1 block)

□ absent (no adipose tissue)

- Infiltration of the excretory tract

□ yes

□ no

□ absent (no excretory tracts found)

- Minimum margin for surgical excision (inked)

□ **damage**

□ **healthy I__I__I mm (>>1 block)**

F- Removing the tumor :

- Full inclusion for small tumors (<2 cm)
- If the lesion is too large to be included in its entirety:

- 1 block per cm of longest tumor axis

- Including tumor reports (*)

- With the renal capsule, peri-renal fat and excretory tracts.

- Including minimum margins for excision

- Deep (inked surgical section slice)
- Lateral (perirenal adipose tissue)

I - Necessary equipment

- Fixing agent: The usual fixing agent is 10% buffered formalin.
- blade
- Knife
- Indian ink
- Flat ruler
- Tapes
- Camera

K. Conditions and rules of good practice

- Parts are fixed in 10% buffered formalin.
- Delayed or poor fixation can alter the morphological quality of histological sections. It is important to respect the ratio of tissue volume to fixative volume (1/10).

- All specimens must be accompanied by a **clinical information sheet**. This sheet should include the history of the disease, the patient's background, the results of any paraclinical examinations carried out, and endoscopic data.

K. Conclusion

In conclusion, a methodical and accurate approach to the macroscopic examination of nephrectomy specimens is imperative to characterize tumor lesions, assess resection margins and provide crucial information for patient prognosis and management. By following the guidelines presented in this guide, pathology professionals will be able to perfect their ability to accurately interpret the macroscopic characteristics of tumors, thus contributing to more effective, individualized patient management.

What to sample

- **Tumor**

Full inclusion if tumor small (<2cm)

If the lesion cannot be included in its entirety :

1 block per cm of longest tumor axis

- **Reports (if any)**

Tumor/kidney capsule ratio

Ratio of tumor to perirenal adipose tissue

Tumor to excretory tract ratio

- **Minimum margin for surgical excision**

Minimum margin for deep surgical excision

Minimal margin for lateral surgical excision

(Peri-renal adipose tissue)

TOTAL NEPHRECTOMY

TOTAL NEPHRECTOMY

A- Inking, kidney description :

- **Fram**

In most cases, inking is not necessary. Ink if necessary:

- Peripheral indurated zones
- The external surface of the tumor if there is no fat.

- **Weigh** the entire surgical specimen

I__I__I__I__Igrams

- **Measure** the kidney in all 3 dimensions

I__I__I__Ix I__I__I__Ix I__I__Imm

B- Ureter :

- **Locating** the ureter
- **Measuring** the ureter

I__I__I__Imm

- Distal ureteral limit **sampling** (1 block)
- **Catheterize** the ureter retrogradely from the ureteral border into the renal pelvis before opening the specimen.

C- Opening the room :

Opening on a coronal plane

- Do not uncap the kidney

- Open the part vertically in a frontal cutting plane, defined by the stylus, from the outer edge to the inner edge (renal hilum).

D- Part orientation :

- **Adrenal:** orange-yellow, at the upper pole of the kidney, extending over the upper part of the medial border.
- **In case of tumor:** (here upper pole) Check if tumor location corresponds to clinical information

Renal hilum: medial

Ureter: Path from pyelon to lower pole

It runs along the medial edge of the kidney to its lower pole.

Easily found before opening, its end corresponding to the lower-medial part of the kidney.

E- Renal vein :

- **Specify if there is a tumor thrombus in the renal vein** (arrow)

□ yes□ no

N.B.: in the case of thrombus, it may be useful to include the vascular border of the renal pedicle (1 block).

- Otherwise systematically include 1 vascular hilum block comprising renal artery and vein

F- Adrenal :

- **Adrenal gland**

□ yes (enlarged nephrectomy) □ no

- **Measuring** its longest axis

I__I__I__Imm

- **Weighing** the adrenal gland

I__I__I__I__Igrams

- **Nodules** o yes o no

if so, specify their relationship to the tumor

- **Sampling of** the adrenal gland and its relationship to the tumour (1 block and more if lesional)

G- Tumor location

- Check that tumour location is superimposable on clinical information.

- Specify **the initial site of the tumor**:
  - □ Parenchymal
  - □ Excretory pathways

- Specify the **location of** the tumor:
  - □ Upper fleece
  - □ Median kidney
  - □ Bottom polar
  - □ Hilaire
  - □ Massive

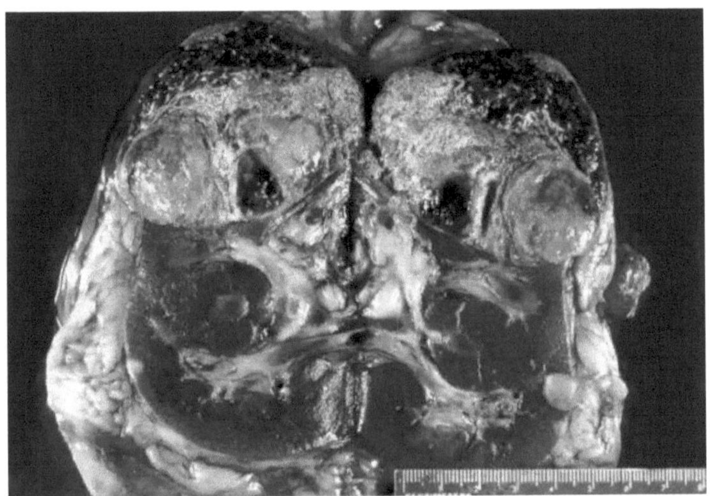

Figure 1: Tumor of the upper pole of the kidney

https://www.webpathology.com/images/genitourinary/kidney/renal-cell-carcinomas---i/35860...

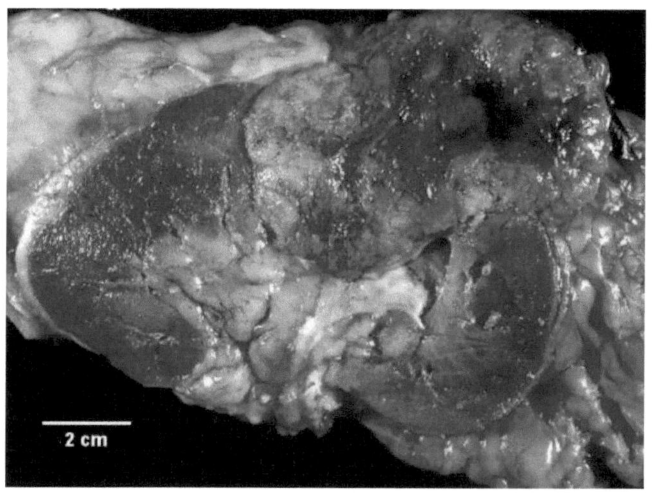

Figure 2: Mid-renal tumor

https://www.webpathology.com/images/genitourinary/kidney/renal-cell-carcinomas---i/35859.

H- Description of the tumor :

- **Measuring** the tumor:

I__I__I__Ix I__I__I__Ix I__I__Imm

- Assessing its **contours** :

□ Well limited□ Poorly limited

□ Encapsulated□ Non-encapsulated

- Evaluate its **consistency** :

□ Farm

□ Soft

- Describe its **color**

□ Chamois yellow

□ Light beige

□ mahogany brown

□ polychrome or other

- Describe the **remodeling** :

□ necrotic: I__I__I %.

□ bleeding

□ scarring

I- Tumor samples :

- **Full inclusion** if tumor small (< 2 cm)

- **Take 1 block per cm of the longest axis of** the tumour (if > 2 cm), giving priority to the **various ratios**:

- with the **renal capsule**: o involved o distant I__I__I)mm) (1 block)

- with **peri-renal fat**: o infiltrated (depth I__I__I mm) o healthy 1 block)

- with the **renal hilum**: o infiltrated o healthy (2 blocks with vessels)

- with **excretory tracts**: Calyx invasion o yes o no

Basin invasion o yes o no (1 block)

J- Lymph nodes :

Macroscopic examination reveals lymph nodes only inconstantly.

- Palpate for sinus **adenopathy**

- **Include all lymph nodes** found

K- Non-tumoral kidney

- Harvest **normal peri-tumoral kidney** at tumor junction (1 block)

- Remove the **normal kidney at a distance** from the tumour (1 to 2 blocks)

- **Check for lesions**

- parenchymal (o cyst, o tumor)

- urinary tract

In particular, look for a synchronous parenchymal tumor lesion, which is not exceptional.

I - Necessary equipment

- Fixing agent: The usual fixing agent is 10% buffered formalin.
- blade
- Knife
- India ink
- Flat ruler
- Tapes
- Camera

L. Conditions and rules of good practice

- Parts are fixed in 10% buffered formalin.
- Delayed or poor fixation can alter the morphological quality of histological sections. It is important to respect the ratio of tissue volume to fixative volume (1/10).

- All specimens must be accompanied by a **clinical information sheet**. This sheet should include the history of the disease, the patient's background, the results of any paraclinical examinations carried out, and endoscopic data.

K. Conclusion

In conclusion, a methodical and accurate approach to the macroscopic examination of nephrectomy specimens is imperative to characterize tumor lesions, assess resection margins and provide crucial information for patient prognosis and management. By following the guidelines presented in this guide, pathology professionals will be able to perfect their ability to accurately interpret the macroscopic characteristics of tumors, thus contributing to more effective, individualized patient management.

What to sample

Ten to fifteen blocks are usually taken in the following order:

1. **Distal ureteral limit** (1 block)

2. **Adrenal**: (1 block if healthy, 2 or more if tumorous)

3. **Sinus (vascular hilum)**: (2 or 3 blocks) containing the renal artery and vein and possibly a thrombus

macroscopic renal vein - **vascular border**

4. **Tumor and its relationships** (1 block per cm of tumor)

- **tumor/renal hilum** ratio
- **tumor/kidney** capsule ratio
- ratio of tumor to **fat**
- ratio of tumor to **pyelocal cavities**

5. **hilar lymph nodes**

6. **Non-tumoral renal parenchyma :**

- normal peritumoral kidney (1block)
- normal remote kidney (1block)

7. **Any** suspected parenchymal or urinary tract **lesion**

NEPHRECTOMY FOR EXCRETORY TRACT TUMOR

NEPHRECTOMY FOR EXCRETORY TRACT TUMOR

A- Frame / Measure / Weigh

- In the absence of visible tumor extension, there is no need to ink the specimen.

- **Measure** the kidney in its 3 axes I__I__I__Ix I__I__I__Ix I__I__Imm

- **Weigh** the entire kidney: I__I__I__I__I grams

B- Sampling the ureteral limit

- **Locating** the ureter

- **Measure** its length I__I__I__I mm

- Ureteral limit **sampling** (1 block)

- Then catheterize the ureter to open the room

C- Opening the room:

Retrograde ureter catheterization

- Do not uncap the kidney.

- Pass a stylet (or probe) through the ureter and up into the renal pelvis.

- Open the part vertically in a frontal cutting plane, defined by the stylus, from the outer edge to the inner edge (renal hilum).

D- Orient the part:

Adrenal: (absent here) orange-yellow, upper pole of kidney and upper part of medial border.

In case of tumour: check that the location corresponds to the clinical information

Renal hilum: medio-renal and medial position

Ureter: from the pyelon to the lower pole, runs along the lower part of the medial border of the kidney to its lower pole

E- Adrenal :

- Adrenal: o yes (enlarged nephrectomy) o no

- Measure its longest axis: I__I__I__I mm

- Weigh the adrenal gland: I__I__I__I grams

- Weigh kidney without adrenals: I__I__I__I__I__I grams

- Nodule(s): o yes o no if yes, specify relationship to tumour

- Sampling of the adrenal gland and its relationship to the tumour (1 block and more if lesional)

F- Description of the tumor :

- Location

Superimposable on clinical information?

□ Calyx o upper o middle o lower

□ Pyélon (ex- bassinet)

□ Pyeloureteral junction

□ Ureter

- Measuring the tumor:

I__I__I__Ix I__I__I__Ix I__I__Imm

- Contours :

□ well limited o poorly limited

□ papillary o non papillary

□ infiltrating o non-infiltrating

- Take 1 block per cm of tumour with the following ratios

G- Specify relationships :

- Infiltration of the wall of the excretory tract:

□ yes (depth: I__I__I mm)

□ no (1 block)

- Infiltration of the renal parenchyma :

□ yes (depth: I__I__I mm)

□ no (margin : I__I__I mm) (1 block)

- Infiltration of the hilum:

□ yes

□ no (margin : I__I__I mm) (1 block)

- Distance tumor recuts ureter I__I__I__I mm

H- Look for synchronous lesions of the excretory tract

· **Search for distant synchronous tumor localization**

· Describe excretory tract and parenchymal changes resulting from the tumor (hydronephrosis, ureteral dilatation, etc.).

· Remove any suspicious lesion

I- Look for adenopathy in the hilum :

- On palpation.
- Include all nodes found.

Macroscopic examination reveals lymph nodes only inconstantly.

J- Non-tumoral kidney :

- Normal peritumoral kidney at tumor junction (1 block)
- Normal kidney away from tumor (1 block)
- Check for parenchymal lesions (cysts, etc.). If necessary, take

K - Necessary equipment

- Fixing agent: The usual fixing agent is 10% buffered formalin.
- blade
- Knife
- Indian ink
- Flat ruler
- Tapes
- Camera

Conditions and rules of good practice

- Parts are fixed in 10% buffered formalin.
- Delayed or poor fixation can alter the morphological quality of histological sections. It is important to respect the ratio of tissue volume to fixative volume (1/10).

- All specimens must be accompanied by a **clinical information sheet**. This sheet should include the history of the disease, the patient's background, the results of any paraclinical examinations carried out, and endoscopic data.

M. Conclusion

In conclusion, a methodical and accurate approach to the macroscopic examination of nephrectomy specimens is imperative to characterize tumor lesions, assess resection margins and provide crucial information for patient prognosis and management. By following the guidelines presented in this guide, pathology professionals will be able to perfect their ability to accurately interpret the macroscopic characteristics of tumors, thus contributing to more effective, individualized patient management.

What to sample

Include in the following order

Ureteral/ureteral **boundary** (1 block)

Adrenal gland (1 block if healthy, more if tumorous)

The tumor (1 block/cm) **and its relationships :**

Relationship with the wall of the excretory tract (maximum infiltration)

Ratio and infiltration of renal parenchyma

Renal hilum ratio and infiltration

Any lymph nodes in the renal hilum

Non-tumoral renal parenchyma

Normal peritumoral kidney (1 block)

Remote normal kidney (1 block)

Any synchronous lesion of the upper urinary tract

Any suspected parenchymal lesion

TESTICULE

TESTICULE

A- Description of the testis :

- An even, oblong organ located in the **scrotum**.
- Surrounded by a thick (1mm) fibrous shell: the **albuginea**.
- It consists of **seminiferous tubules** organized into lobules separated by fibrous septa. Spermatozoa are excreted from these tubes. These are followed by the straight tubes, which collect in the **rete testis**, then in the **epididymis** and **vas deferens**, before joining the urinary tract at the prostatic urethra.
- Between the seminiferous tubules, Leydig cells secrete testosterone.
- **Average total weight** (adult): 14-20 grams
- **Average size** (in an adult): 4 cm long by 2.5 cm thick by 3 cm anterior-posterior diameter.

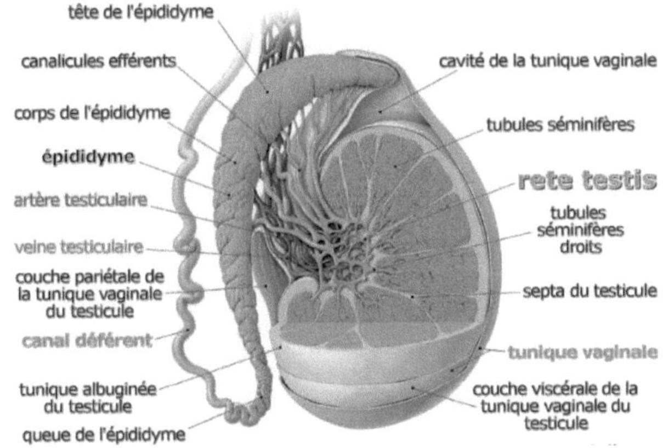

Figure 1: Diagram of a testicle

https://www.aquaportail.com/dictionnaire/definition/3367/testicule

B- Its reports :

- It is surrounded by a **testicular vagina**, with the exception of its posterior edge and lower part.
- The **epididymis** drains the rete testis at its head at the upper pole of the testis, then descends reflecting on the posterior edge of the testis to form the body and tail.

- It separates at the middle part of the testicle, where it is called the **vas deferens**, and then ascends to the prostate.

C- Orientation criteria :

There are no reliable landmarks for macroscopically distinguishing between right and left orchiectomy.

- The **spermatic cord** (vas deferens) comes into contact with the testicle at its posteroinferior part.
- The head of **the epididymis** is located at the upper pole of the testicle.
- The epididymis runs along the posterior edge of the testicle.
- The **vagina** encircles the testicle

Except for the posterior edge and lower part of the testicle.

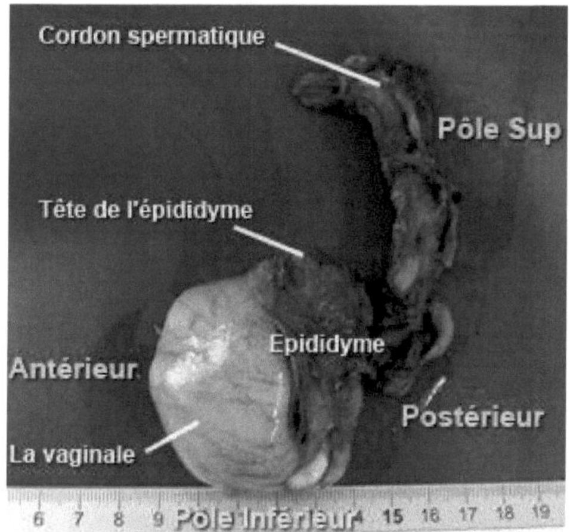

Figure 2: Criteria for orienting an orchiectomy specimen

D- Measurement

- Measuring **the cord**

I__I__I__Imm

- Measure the **testicle** in all three axes

I__I__Ix I__I__I x I__I__I mm

E- Cord sampling :

It is important to remove the spermatic cord **before opening the orchiectomy specimen**, to avoid contamination of the spermatic cord, and to avoid over-grafting the tumor with false emboli.

Detach the cord, then take 3 cross-sectional levels in the following order:

- **distal** section slice (surgical limit) (1 block)

- **medium-section** slice (1 block)

- **proximal** section slice (juxta-testicular part) (1 block)

F- Inking :

Inking is not usually necessary for orchidectomy parts.

Vaginal opening

Section the vagina, if present, by its anterior side.

Note the presence of any hydrocele (liquid effusion from the testicular vagina).

□ yes□ no

G- Testicular section :

Section the testicle **along its longest axis** (sagittal axis)

2 possibilities :

➔ **Opening in the fresh state,** initially respecting the epididymis in order to make subsequent cuts passing through the epididymis after fixation

➔ **Opening after fixation,** opening via the epididymis

H- Testicular weighing :

Weighing the testicle

I__I__I__Igrams

I- Description of the tumor and the non-tumoral testis :

☐ Photograph the open room

☐ Description of **tumor**

- **Number of** tumor nodules
- Tumor measurement in all 3 axes

■ **Appearance**: **necrosis %**, heterogeneity, consistency, remodelling (haemorrhages, cysts, mucoid territories, fibrosis, calcifications or ossifications)

■ **Note ratios and margins**

→ With albuginea

→ With the epididymis

→ With cord

■ **Description of the non-tumoral testis**

- Fibrous appearance
- Presence of accessory nodules

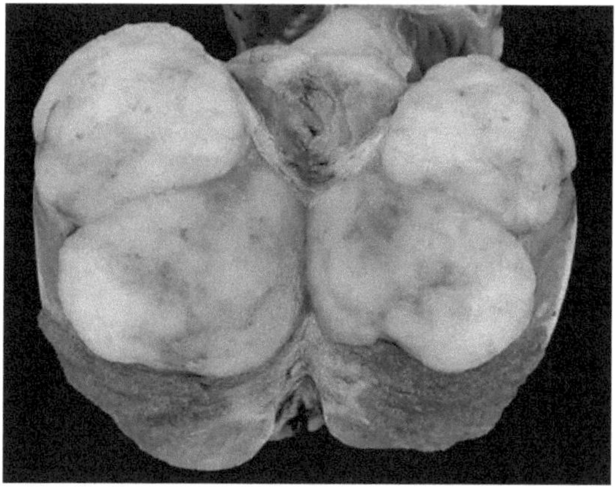

Figure 3: Whitish, multinodular, sharply demarcated testicular tumor.

https://www.webpathology.com/images/genitourinary/testis/germ-cell-tumors---i/36454.

J- Removal of tumor and non-tumor testis :

- **Small tumors 1 to 2 cm in size**: fully included

- **Tumors larger than 2 cm :**

Include at least 1 block per cm of longest tumour axis.
Sampling **macroscopically areas**

- Necrotic and hemorrhagic zones
- areas

Take **reports** with

- With albuginea (1 block)
- With the epididymis (head and posterior surface) (1 to 2 blocks)
- With the emergence of the cord (1 block)

- Non-tumoral testis and epididymis:

Normal testicle: normal testicle - tumor relationships (2 blocks)

Epididymi

- testicle-epididymis relationship (head and posterior surface) (2 blocks)

- epididymal-tumoral relationship if possible

K - equipment

- Fixing agent: The usual fixing agent is 10% buffered formalin.
- blade
- Knife
- Indian ink
- Flat ruler
- Tapes
- Camera

L. Conditions and rules of good practice

- Parts are fixed in 10% buffered formalin.
- Delayed or poor fixation can alter the morphological quality of histological sections. It is important to respect the ratio of tissue volume to fixative volume (1/10).

- All specimens must be accompanied by a **clinical information sheet**. This sheet should include the history of the disease, the patient's background, the results of any paraclinical examinations carried out, and endoscopic data.

M. Conclusion

In conclusion, a methodical and accurate approach to macroscopic examination of orchiectomy specimens is imperative to characterize tumor lesions, assess resection margins and provide crucial information for prognosis and patient management.

By following the guidelines presented in this guide, anatomical pathology professionals will be able to perfect their ability to accurately interpret the macroscopic features of tumors, thus contributing to more effective, individualized patient management.

What to sample

▪ Spermatic cord

Always first before sectioning the testicle

- Distal section slice (surgical limit) (1 block)
- Medium-section slice (1 block)
- Proximal section slice (juxta testicular part) (1 block)

▪ Tumor

· **Small tumors 1 to 2 cm:** include all tumors

· **Tumors larger than 2 cm**

Include at least 1 block per cm of longest tumour axis.

Sampling macroscopically areas

- Necrotic and hemorrhagic zones
- areas

Take reports

- With albuginea (1 block)
- With the epididymis (head and posterior surface) (1 to 2 blocks)
- With cord (1 block)

▪ Non-tumoral testis and epididymis

· **Normal testicle**: normal testicle - tumor relationships (2 blocks)

- Testicular-epididymal relationship (head and posterior surface) (2 blocks)
- Epididymis-tumor ratio if possible

CYSTO-PROSTATECTOMY

CYSTO-PROSTATECTOMY

A- Anatomy - orientation :

1- Bladder :

The bladder derives embryologically from the urogenital sinus.
The bladder is a cavity/reservoir at the confluence of the upper excretory tracts (right and left ureters) and its shape varies according to its replenishment.
Urine escapes through the urethra opposite the bladder neck.

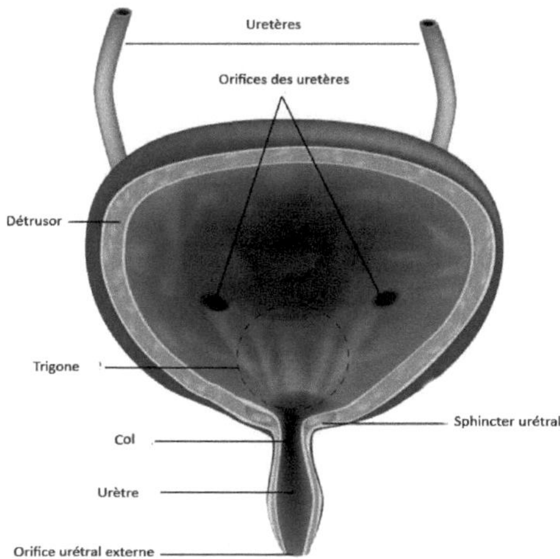

Figure 1: Diagram illustrating the bladder

https://cancer-parc-tubiana.docvitae.fr/cancer-de-la-vessie-et-des-voies-urinaires/la-vessie-un-schema-pour-comprendre

2- Bladder wall :

- **The urothelium** lines the bladder cavity containing the urine.

- **A muscular mucosa** divides the sub-epithelial connective tissue into **superficial** and **deep chorion**.
- The thick muscularis is also called **detrusor** at bladder level.
- **Peri-vesical adipose tissue** comprises a peritonealized portion (upper surface and posterior part) and a non-peritonealized portion corresponding to the surgical removal path (to be inked).

3- Different bladder regions :

The trigone is the triangular area of the posterior surface between the ureteral orifices and the bladder neck.

Here, **the anterior surface** is cut to open the bladder.

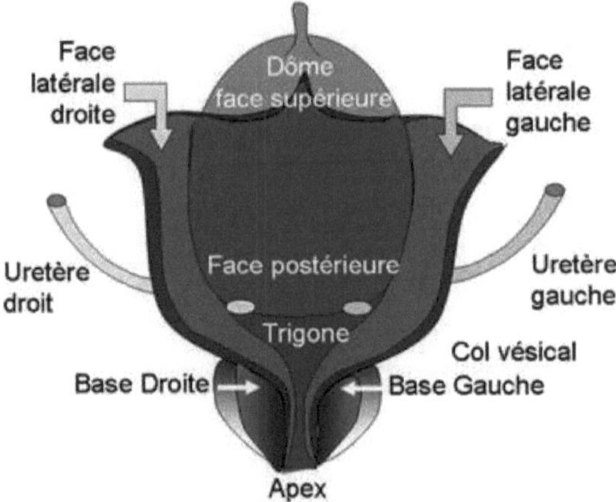

Figure 2: Different bladder regions

4- Prostate :

The prostate is at the junction of the urinary (urethra) and spermatic (vas deferens) ducts.

The prostatic urethra runs from the base (upwards and forwards) to the apex (downwards and backwards).

It is joined in the middle by the ejaculatory ducts, which cross the prostate from the posterior-superior part.

Several authors have attempted to describe the prostatic regions

The anatomical description describes :

- the **isthmus** in front of the urethra.

- the **middle lobe** between the urethra at the front and the ejaculatory ducts at the back

- the **right and left prostatic lobes** behind the ejaculatory ducts on either side of the middle lobe.

The histological description (Mc Neal) describes four regions

- the central zone: surrounds the vas deferens, with the posterosuperior base of the cone forming the base of the prostate.

- the transitional zone: located around the proximal part of the prostatic urethra. For some authors, it belongs to the peripheral zone.

- the peripheral zone: (70% of the prostate) surrounds the central and transitional zones at the top of the prostate and the entire distal prostatic urethra below the veru montanum.

- the anterior fibromuscular zone: devoid of prostate glands, it lines the anterior surface of the prostate, giving it its convex appearance.

Average total weight: 20 grams

Average size: 3cm high, 4cm wide and 2cm thick.

5- Peritoneum

The peritoneum (green dotted line) covers the upper part of the bladder and descends posteriorly to form the cul de sac of Douglas.

The macroscopic appearance is smooth and shiny

6- Local regional reports :

The bladder responds

- forward to the **abdominal wall** and **symphysis pubis**
- back to the **rectum** and **seminal vesicles**
- above the **peritoneal cavity**
- below, opposite the bladder neck to the **prostate**
- lateral to the pelvic sidewalls

7- Orientation criteria :

- **The prostate** is located at the bottom.
- Its anterior surface is convex
- Flat posterior surface.
- **The ureters**, identified by the surgeon using a lake or probe, are located in the posterior part of the specimen.
- **The peritoneum** covers the upper part of the bladder and descends posteriorly to form the cul de sac of Douglas

B- Preparing the part :

· **Surgical part size:** I__I__I__Ix I__I__I__Ix I__I__I__Imm

- **Remove clips** and sutures to avoid tissue tearing, a source of false positive margins

- **Ink the entire surgical part**,

2 different colors available for front and back.

Allow to dry for 5 minutes, dab with paper, then immerse the workpiece for 1 minute in acetic formaldehyde or Bouin, for etching.

C- Open and describe the operating room

- **Catheterize the prostatic urethra** from the prostatic apex to the base (vesical neck and lumen)

- **Cut sagittally** along the stylet in the middle of **the anterior face**.

- **Spread** the edges of the surgical specimen and describe the lesion

- **Photograph** of surgical specimen o yes o no

- **Fix** the surgical specimen for a maximum of 48 hours in buffered formalin/acetic formalin

D- Ureters

- **Measuring**

Right ureter I__I__I__I mm

Left ureter I__I__I__I mm

- Collect right and left ureteral borders if not communicated separately (2 blocks)

- Catheterize the ureters from their proximal limit

Saline can be injected to dilate the ureters.

If the ureters are not found on the external surface, try to catheterize them from the ureteral orifices via the endovesical route.

- Open along the stylets and locate the right and ureteral orifices

- Describe their relationship to the tumor

Tumor - Right ureteral orifice: I__I__Imm

Tumor - Left ureteral orifice: I__I__I mm

- Harvest right and left ureteral orifices 2 blocks)

E- Seminal vesicles :

- Right seminal vesicle size: I__I__I__I mm

- Size of **left** seminal vesicle: I__I__I__I mm

- Infiltration of the seminal vesicles:

o right VS o left VS o no infiltration

- Cutting the seminal vesicle

- 1 base unit

- 1 longitudinal section

Make one block per vesicle (2 blocks)

F- Prostate :

After opening on the front (step 3)

- Prostate size

Height: I__I__I__Imm Width: I__I__Imm Thickness: I__I__Imm

- Locating the bladder neck

Measure distance from **tumor to bladder neck:** I__I__I mm

Remove cone-shaped bladder flange (1 block)

Scalpel notch on left to differentiate laterality under microscopy

- Cut the prostate into **macroscopically serialized horizontal slices.**

Take 5 slices, isolating right and left lobes (10 blocks)

G- Describe the tumor :

- Number of tumors :

□ No visible tumor □ Unique

□ Multifocal (Number:__I__I I)□ Diffuse

- Tumor location(s) :

□ Dome□ Front

□ Ureteral orifice D□ Ureteral orifice G

□ Trigone□ Posterior side

□ Cervix□ Prostatic urethra

□ Side D□ Side G

□ Tumor in

- Tumor size

Main tumor: I__I__I__I x I__I__I__I mm

Maximum infiltration depth: I__I__I mm

Accessory tumors: I__I__I mm, I__I__I mm, I__I__I mm

- Growth mode :

□ budding□ infiltrating□ ulcerated□ unspecified

- Necrotic changes : yes

H- Removing the tumor :

Tumor >5 blocks)

At least 5 blocks at a rate of 1 block per cm, best involving a complete tumor slice with **maximum infiltration depth** and tumor surface.

Infiltration depth :

- mucous membrane□ no□ yes

- muscular (Detrusor) o no o yes

Macroscopically, it is difficult to determine the depth of muscular infiltration (superficial or deep).

- perivesical tissues o no o yes

Reports

margins for surgical excision

With non-peritonealized bank (perivesical tissue)

o reached (location:) o distant I__I__I)mm) (1 block)

with the serosa (peritoneal):

o reached (location:) o distant I__I__I)mm) (1 block)

- **Tumor to non-tumor bladder ratio** (1 block)

I- Harvesting the peri-tumoral bladder:

- **Measure** bladder: I__I__Ix I__I__Ix I__I__I__Imm

- **Describe** the non-tumoral bladder mucosa

o normal o polypoid o fragile o ulcerated o diverticular

- **Non-tumoral bladder mapping** (locate): (up to 6 blocks)

o block trigone:I__I__I

o block dome:I__I__I

o anterior face block:I__I__I

o posterior face block:I__I__I

o right lateral face block:I__I__I

o left side block:I__I__I

- **Peri-vesical structures**

Nodules in peri-vesical adipose tissue

Number:

Long axis of the largest: I__I__I mm

I - Necessary equipment

- Fixing agent: The usual fixing agent is 10% buffered formalin.
- blade
- Knife
- India ink
- Flat ruler
- Tapes
- Camera

B. Conditions and rules of good practice

- Parts are fixed in 10% buffered formalin.
- Delayed or poor fixation can alter the morphological quality of histological sections. It is important to respect the ratio of tissue volume to fixative volume (1/10).

- All specimens must be accompanied by a **clinical information sheet**. This sheet should include the history of the disease, the patient's background, the results of any paraclinical examinations carried out, and endoscopic data.

K. Conclusion

In conclusion, a methodical and accurate approach to the macroscopic examination of radical cystoprostatectomy specimens is imperative to characterize tumor lesions, assess resection margins and provide crucial information for patient prognosis and management. By following the guidelines presented in this guide, pathology professionals will be able to perfect their ability to accurately interpret the macroscopic characteristics of tumors, thus contributing to more effective, individualized patient management.

What to sample

■ Limits
- Left and right ureteral borders (2 blocks)
- Right ureteral orifice (1 block)
- Left ureteral orifice (1 block)
- Bladder flange (cone-shaped) (1 block)

■ Seminal vesicles
- 1 block per seminal vesicle (2 blocks)

■ Prostate
5 macroscopic slices from apex to base, isolating right and left (10 blocks)
By locating the posterior part through an incision
For suspected prostate lesions: refer to protocol

■ Tumor
At least 5 blocks at a rate of 1 block per cm (>5 blocks)
A complete tumor slice with the **zone of maximum infiltration** and the **tumor surface** is of greatest interest

■ Tumor relationships
The **margin with the inked, non-peritoneal surgical excision margin** of the peri-vesical tissues corresponding to the minimal surgical excision (locate)
The **margin with the serosa** (non-inked peritoneal zone)
Tumor to non-tumor **bladder** ratio

■ Non-tumoral bladder
- Non-tumoral bladder mapping (locate): (up to 6 blocks)
Trigon, dome, front, back, right and left sides
Peri-vesical structures :
Nodules in peri-vesical adipose tissue

PROSTATE

Prostate

A- Orientation criteria :

To orientate the surgical specimen, pass a **stylet** through the urethra: the urethra is median at the apex and anterior at the base.

The base is at the top.

The **seminal vesicles** are located superiorly and posteriorly.

The posterior, **rectal surface** is flat, while the anterior surface is convex.

The pointed **apex** is at the bottom.

B- Inking

- **Remove sutures** and clips to avoid tissue tearing, a source of false positive margins

- **Ink** the entire surgical specimen, including the seminal vesicles (2 colors D and G if necessary)

- **Allow to dry** for 5 minutes, then immerse the workpiece (1 to 2 minutes) in acetic formaldehyde or white vinegar, to mordant the Indian ink, before fixing with 10% formaldehyde or acetic formaldehyde.

C- Measurement - Weighing :

Prostate :

- Height: apex to base

- Width (transverse diameter)

- Prostate thickness: anteroposterior diameter.

Seminal vesicles :

Measure the right and left seminal vesicles along their longest axis.

Weigh the prostate before and after removal of the seminal vesicles.

Weigh seminal vesicles

The surgical specimen must be inked before the seminal vesicles are detached

D- Fixing :

- In 10% formalin or **acetic formalin**.

- Fixation time: 24 h if pre-cut or small prostate; **48 to 60 h** if unopened or large part.

- Pre-cutting into thick slices (2 cm thick with a maximum of 2 slices to avoid deforming the part), perpendicular to the urethra and rectal surface, is possible, enabling faster fixation.

E- Bladder neck sampling

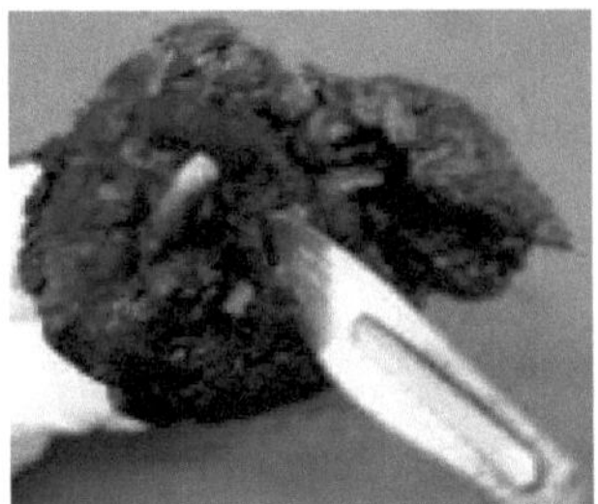

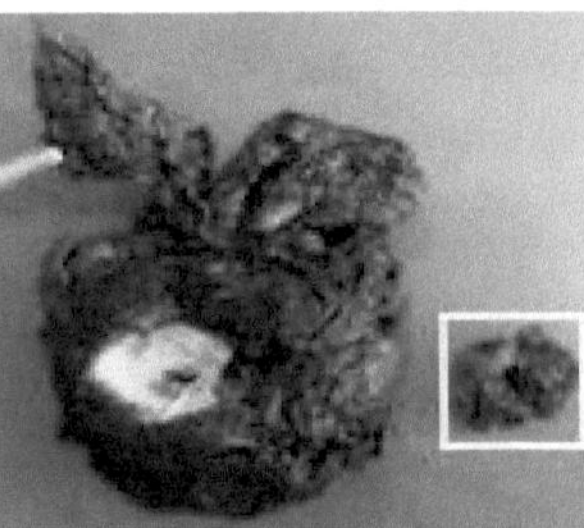

Figure 2: Bladder neck sampling

1 Isolating the cervix: Removing a cone from around the stylet on the upper surface, perpendicular to the cervix.

urethra (2 mm thick)

F- Seminal vesicle sampling

G- Base withdrawal :

Base sampling (proximal or upper surgical margin)

Full inclusion of the sagittal sections of the base. **Blocks A**

A horizontal slice of the base, 3 to 6 mm thick, is cut sagittally to the right and left, working from the center outwards.

H- Apex sampling :

Apex harvesting (distal or inferior surgical margin)

- Full inclusion of sagittal sections of the apex. **C blocks**
- A horizontal slice of the apex, 3 to 6 mm thick, with sagittal cuts, distinguishing right and left apexes.
- Ex CD (right) and CG (left) blocks. The inner side of the cuts faces the bottom of the cassette. A posterior notch can be made.

I- Cross-sectional sampling of the prostate gland

Staged transverse sections of the entire gland, perpendicular to the rectal surface and urethra: 2-3 mm thick sections, from apex to base. Each slice is identified by a letter from E to X.

The sections are included in their entirety, separating the right and left sides. The posterior surface is incised for better orientation on the sections.

Right side, left side and front part separation, if it does not fit into the cassette.

In the case of a large surgical specimen, if it is not possible to include the entire prostate, place the entire specimen in numbered cassettes and include only one slice out of 2. These cassettes can be included secondarily if no tumour proliferation is found on the blocks initially included.

What to describe?

- **Size**: - prostate height, width, thickness

  - length of seminal vesicles

- **Weight**: - prostate with seminal vesicles

  - seminal vesicles

  - prostate without seminal vesicles

- **Lesions** of the prostate are generally not visible macroscopically, which is why it is necessary to include the entire gland.

J - Necessary equipment

- Fixing agent: The usual fixing agent is 10% buffered formalin.
- blade
- Knife
- Indian ink
- Flat ruler
- Tapes
- Camera

K. Conditions and rules of good practice

- Parts are fixed in 10% buffered formalin.
- Delayed or poor fixation can alter the morphological quality of histological sections. It is important to respect the ratio of tissue volume to fixative volume (1/10).
- All specimens must be accompanied by a **clinical information sheet**. This sheet should include the history of the disease, the patient's background, the results of any paraclinical examinations carried out, and endoscopic data.

L. Conclusion

In conclusion, a methodical and accurate approach to the macroscopic examination of prostatectomy specimens is imperative to characterize tumor lesions, assess resection margins and provide crucial information for patient prognosis and management. By following the guidelines presented in this guide, pathology professionals will be able to perfect their ability to accurately interpret the macroscopic characteristics of tumors, thus contributing to more effective, individualized patient management.

What to sample

Prostate sampling is systematized according to the modified Mac Neal technique. **The entire prostate must be included**.

Note: in Mac Neal's technique, section B (bladder neck) is taped first, followed by section D (seminal vesicles), then section A (base) and finally section C (apex).

In order

- B block: bladder neck

- DD and DG blocks: seminal vesicles

- AD and AG blocks: base

- CD and CG blocks: apex

- ED, EG +/- EA blocks: first slice near the apex

- blocks FD, FG +/- F1: second macroscopic slice from bottom to top

- blocks G, H, ... include all slices from apex to base

If the prostate is too large, every second macroscopic slice can be included, with the slices not included kept on numbered cassettes.

CONCLUSION

In conclusion, this Practical Guide to Urological Pathology is an essential reference for anatomopathologists faced with the meticulous examination of urological surgical specimens. By highlighting the subtleties of macroscopic analysis, this book offers a rigorous methodology and protocols for the accurate interpretation of specific pathologies of the urogenital tract, particularly malignant forms.

This guide, designed to provide enlightened guidance for diagnostic and therapeutic practices, is intended to be an indispensable companion in the acquisition of the knowledge required for advanced expertise in urological pathological anatomy. Each specimen thus becomes a source of in-depth learning, enabling precise identification of lesions, meticulous description, and evaluation of prognostic markers crucial to optimal patient management.

By encouraging an analytical and critical approach to each case, this book aspires to nurture the intellectual curiosity and professionalism of practitioners, inspiring them to pursue a relentless quest for self-improvement. May this resource become the pillar of your practice, propelling your expertise to new heights and contributing to the ongoing advancement of urological medicine.

SUMMARY

This guide is aimed at specialists training in pathological anatomy and focuses on the macroscopic examination of urological surgical specimens. It covers nephrectomy specimens, excretory tract tumors, testicular specimens, cystoprostatectomies and radical prostatectomies. The guide offers clear protocols for tumor identification and description, with an emphasis on essential prognostic factors. Its aim is to enhance specialists' skills and improve the quality of diagnosis in urological pathology.

BIBLIOGRAPHICAL REFERENCES

1. Varma M, Dormer J. Macroscopy of specimens from the genitourinary system. Clin Pathol. 2024;77(3):177-183.

2. Daniel L, Liprandi A, De Fromont M, Lechevallier E, Pellissier JF. General principles of macroscopic examination of kidney tumors. Annales de Pathologie. 1998;18(2):152.

3. Drabent P, Picard C, Dijoud F, Galmiche L, Mussini C, Boudjemaa S, Coulomb-L'Hermine A, Berrebi D. Macroscopic management of nephrectomy surgical specimens after chemotherapy for pediatric kidney tumors. Revue Francophone des Laboratoires. 2022;538:30-37.

4. Varma M, Collins LC, Chetty R, Karamchandani DM, Talia K, Dormer J, Vyas M, Conn B, Guzmán-Arocho YD, Jones AV, Pring M, McCluggage WG. Macroscopic examination of pathology specimens: a critical reappraisal. Clin Pathol. 2024;77(3):164-168.

5. https://www.webpathology.com/

6. https://librepathology.org/wiki/Orchiectomy_grossing

7. https://www.uclahealth.org/sites/default/files/documents/Orchiectomy%20%28Neoplastic%29%2005.20.2020%20HY.pdf

8. https://voices.uchicago.edu/grosspathology/gu-renal/prostate-prostatectomy/

9. https://www.uclahealth.org/sites/default/files/documents/Radical%20Prostatectomy%2004.15.22.pdf

10. Rao BV, Soni S, Kulkarni B, et al. Grossing and reporting of radical prostatectomy specimens: An evidence-based approach. J Pathol Inform. 2024;5:123-130.

11. Montironi R, Beltran AL, Mazzucchelli R, et al. Handling of Radical Prostatectomy Specimens: Total Embedding with Large-Format Histology. Int J Breast Cancer. 2012 Jul 10;2012:932784. doi: 10.1155/2012/932784.

12. https://documents.cap.org/protocols/cp-malegenital-prostate-radicalprostatectomy-19-4040.pdf

13. Sung MT, Davidson DD, Montironi R, et al. Radical prostatectomy specimen processing: A critical appraisal of sampling methods. Curr Diagn Pathol. 2007;13(6):490-498.

14. https://www.pathology.med.umich.edu/static/apps/cutting/RADICAL_PROSTATECTOMY_Whole_Mount.pdf

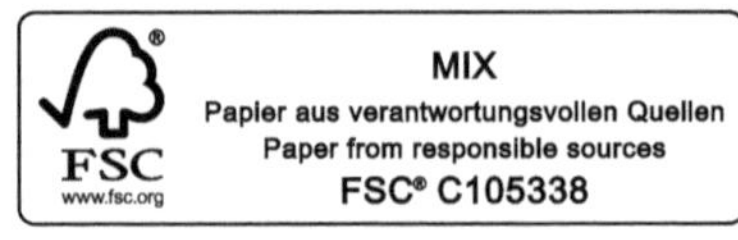

Printed by Books on Demand GmbH, Norderstedt / Germany